THE
PALEO DIET
WORKBOOK

LIVE

LOVE

PALEO

Track Your Progress

Day .... Date..................

- ## Diet Plan

....
....
....

- ## How do you feel?

....
....
....
....

- ## Record your weight: ....

Track Your Progress

Day ....   Date...................

- ## Diet Plan

  ....
  ....
  ....

- ## How do you feel?

  ....
  ....
  ....
  ....

- ## Record your weight: ....

Track Your Progress

Day ....   Date..................

- ## Diet Plan

....
....
....

- ## How do you feel?

....
....
....
....

- ## Record your weight: ....

Track Your Progress

Day ....   **Date**..................

- ### Diet Plan

  ....
  ....
  ....

- ### How do you feel?

  ....
  ....
  ....
  ....

- ### Record your weight: ....

Track Your Progress

Day ....   **Date**..................

- ## Diet Plan

```
..........................................................................
..........................................................................
```

- ## How do you feel?

```
..........................................................................
..........................................................................
..........................................................................
```

- ## Record your weight: ....

<u>Track Your Progress</u>

Day ....   **Date**.................

- ### <u>Diet Plan</u>

  > ....
  >
  > ....

- ### <u>How do you feel?</u>

  > ....
  >
  > ....
  >
  > ....

- ### Record your weight: ....

<u>Track Your Progress</u>

Day ....   **Date**.................

- ## <u>Diet Plan</u>

....

....

....

- ## <u>How do you feel?</u>

....

....

....

....

- ## Record your weight: ....

<u>Track Your Progress</u>

Day ....   **Date**..................

- ### <u>Diet Plan</u>

  ....
  ....
  ....

- ### <u>How do you feel?</u>

  ....
  ....
  ....
  ....

- ### Record your weight: ....

Track Your Progress

Day ....   Date..................

- ## Diet Plan

  ....
  ....
  ....

- ## How do you feel?

  ....
  ....
  ....
  ....

- ## Record your weight: ....

Track Your Progress

Day ....   Date...................

- ## Diet Plan

  ....
  ....

- ## How do you feel?

  ....
  ....
  ....

- ## Record your weight: ....

PALEO WORKBOOK
LIVE **&** LOVE **PALEO**

Track Your Progress

Day ....   **Date**.................

- ### Diet Plan

....
....

- ### How do you feel?

....
....
....

- **Record your weight:** ....

Track Your Progress

Day .... Date..................

- ## Diet Plan

  ....
  ....
  ....

- ## How do you feel?

  ....
  ....
  ....
  ....

- **Record your weight:** ....

Track Your Progress

Day ....   Date..................

- ## Diet Plan

- ## How do you feel?

- ## Record your weight: ....

Track Your Progress

Day .... **Date**.................

- ## Diet Plan

....
....
....

- ## How do you feel?

....
....
....
....

- **Record your weight:** ....

Track Your Progress

Day ....   Date..................

- ## Diet Plan

  ....
  ....
  ....

- ## How do you feel?

  ....
  ....
  ....
  ....

- ## Record your weight: ....

Track Your Progress

Day ....   **Date**..................

- ## Diet Plan

  ....
  ....
  ....

- ## How do you feel?

  ....
  ....
  ....
  ....

- ## Record your weight: ....

Track Your Progress

Day ....   **Date**..................

- ### Diet Plan

....
....
....

- ### How do you feel?

....
....
....
....

- ### Record your weight: ....

Track Your Progress

Day ....   Date.................

- ## Diet Plan

  ....
  ....
  ....

- ## How do you feel?

  ....
  ....
  ....
  ....

- ## Record your weight: ....

Track Your Progress

Day ....   **Date**..................

- ## Diet Plan

  ....
  ....
  ....

- ## How do you feel?

  ....
  ....
  ....
  ....

- ## Record your weight: ....

Track Your Progress

Day ....   **Date**..................

- ## Diet Plan

....
....
....

- ## How do you feel?

....
....
....
....

- ## Record your weight: ....

Track Your Progress

Day ....   Date.................

- ## Diet Plan

....
....
....

- ## How do you feel?

....
....
....
....

- ## Record your weight: ....

<u>Track Your Progress</u>

Day .... **Date**.................

- ## <u>Diet Plan</u>

....
....

- ## <u>How do you feel?</u>

....
....
....

- ## Record your weight: ....

Track Your Progress

Day .... **Date**..................

- ## Diet Plan

- ## How do you feel?

- ## Record your weight: ....

Track Your Progress

Day ....   **Date**.................

- ## Diet Plan

  ....
  ....
  ....

- ## How do you feel?

  ....
  ....
  ....
  ....

- ## Record your weight: ....

Track Your Progress

Day .... Date.................

- ## Diet Plan

  ....
  ....
  ....

- ## How do you feel?

  ....
  ....
  ....
  ....

- ## Record your weight: ....

Track Your Progress

Day ……………………   **Date**………………

- ## Diet Plan

  ```
  ...........................................................
  ...........................................................
  ...........................................................
  ```

- ## How do you feel?

  ```
  ...........................................................
  ...........................................................
  ...........................................................
  ...........................................................
  ```

- **Record your weight:** …………………………

Track Your Progress

Day .... **Date**..................

- ## Diet Plan

....
....

- ## How do you feel?

....
....
....

- **Record your weight:** ....

Track Your Progress

Day .... Date.................

- ## Diet Plan

....
....
....

- ## How do you feel?

....
....
....
....

- **Record your weight:** ....

Track Your Progress

Day .... **Date**.................

- ## Diet Plan

  ....
  ....
  ....

- ## How do you feel?

  ....
  ....
  ....
  ....

- **Record your weight: ....**

Track Your Progress

Day ....   Date................

- ## Diet Plan

....
....
....

- ## How do you feel?

....
....
....
....

- ## Record your weight: ....

Track Your Progress

Day .... Date..................

- ## Diet Plan

- ## How do you feel?

- ## Record your weight: ....

Track Your Progress

Day .... **Date**.................

- ## Diet Plan

....
....

- ## How do you feel?

....
....
....

- ## Record your weight: ....

Track Your Progress

Day ....   **Date**..................

- ## Diet Plan

....
....
....

- ## How do you feel?

....
....
....
....

- **Record your weight:** ....

Track Your Progress

Day ....   **Date**..................

- ## Diet Plan

  ....
  ....
  ....

- ## How do you feel?

  ....
  ....
  ....
  ....

- ## Record your weight: ....

Track Your Progress

Day ....   Date.................

- ## Diet Plan

  ....
  ....

- ## How do you feel?

  ....
  ....
  ....

- ## Record your weight: ....

Track Your Progress

Day .... Date.................

- ## Diet Plan

  ....
  ....
  ....

- ## How do you feel?

  ....
  ....
  ....
  ....

- ## Record your weight: ....

Track Your Progress

Day ....   Date..................

- ### Diet Plan

  ....
  ....
  ....

- ### How do you feel?

  ....
  ....
  ....
  ....

- ### Record your weight: ....

Track Your Progress

Day .... Date..................

- ### Diet Plan

....
....
....

- ### How do you feel?

....
....
....
....

- ### Record your weight: ....

Track Your Progress

Day ....   **Date**.................

- ## Diet Plan

....

....

....

- ## How do you feel?

....

....

....

....

- **Record your weight: ....**

Track Your Progress

Day .... **Date**.................

- ## Diet Plan

....
....
....

- ## How do you feel?

....
....
....
....

- ## Record your weight: ....

Track Your Progress

Day .... **Date**..................

- ### Diet Plan

  ....
  ....

- ### How do you feel?

  ....
  ....
  ....

- **Record your weight:** ....

Track Your Progress

Day .... Date..................

- ## Diet Plan

  ....
  ....
  ....

- ## How do you feel?

  ....
  ....
  ....
  ....

- ## Record your weight: ....

Track Your Progress

Day .... **Date**.................

- ## Diet Plan

....
....
....

- ## How do you feel?

....
....
....
....

- ## Record your weight: ....

Track Your Progress

Day ....   Date.................

- ## Diet Plan

  ....
  ....
  ....

- ## How do you feel?

  ....
  ....
  ....
  ....

- ## Record your weight: ....

Track Your Progress

Day ....   **Date**.................

- ## Diet Plan

....

....

- ## How do you feel?

....

....

....

- ## Record your weight: ....

Track Your Progress

Day .... **Date**.................

- **Diet Plan**

- **How do you feel?**

- **Record your weight:** ....

Track Your Progress

Day ....   **Date**.................

- ## Diet Plan

....

....

....

- ## How do you feel?

....

....

....

....

- **Record your weight: ....**

Track Your Progress

Day ....   Date.................

- ## Diet Plan

  ....
  ....
  ....

- ## How do you feel?

  ....
  ....
  ....
  ....

- ## Record your weight: ....

LIVE

LOVE

PALEO